Essential First Aid Manual

Critical Life-Saving Techniques for Emergencies

Kyle M. Francois, EMT-P, MPH

© 2024 by Kyle M. Francois, EMT-P, MPH
All rights reserved.

No part of this publication may be reproduced, distributed, or transmitted in any form or by any means, including photocopying, recording, or other electronic or mechanical methods, without prior written permission from the publisher, except in the case of brief quotations for reviews or educational purposes.

Disclaimer

This book is intended to serve as a practical resource for individuals, health workers, providers, first responders, and emergency responders seeking to enhance their knowledge of first aid techniques. While every effort has been made to ensure the accuracy and reliability of the information provided, the author and publisher do not guarantee the completeness, applicability, or effectiveness of the techniques in every situation.

The content of this book should not replace professional medical training or advice. Emergency situations can vary greatly, and readers are encouraged to seek guidance from qualified healthcare professionals or attend certified training programs for hands-on experience and advanced skills.

The author and publisher disclaim any responsibility for errors, omissions, or any outcomes resulting from the use or misuse of the information provided herein. The reader assumes full responsibility for their actions and decisions when applying the techniques described in this book.

Acknowledgements

I would like to express my sincere gratitude to all those who have contributed to the completion of Essential First Aid Manual: Critical Life-Saving Techniques for Emergencies.

First and foremost, I thank my family for their unwavering support and encouragement throughout this journey. A special thanks to my colleagues in the emergency medical services field for their valuable insights and experiences, which have greatly enriched the content of this book.

I am also deeply appreciative of the many patients and first responders who have inspired me through their resilience and commitment to life-saving care.

Lastly, I would like to acknowledge my mentors and the countless healthcare professionals whose dedication to advancing emergency care has motivated me to share this knowledge.

This book is dedicated to those who provide critical care in moments of need, and to those who seek to learn and improve the first aid skills that can save lives.

Kyle M. Francois, EMT-P, MPH

Preface

Emergencies happen when we least expect them. Whether it is a car accident, a sudden medical crisis, or a natural disaster, the ability to act swiftly and effectively can mean the difference between life and death. **Essential First Aid Manual: Critical Life-Saving Techniques for Emergencies** was born from the recognition that everyone—from healthcare providers and first responders to laypersons—needs a reliable resource to equip them with the essential skills to manage critical situations.

In my career as an Emergency Medical Technician-Paramedic (EMT-P) and public health professional (MPH), I have witnessed firsthand the pivotal role first aid plays in saving lives. Whether on the front lines of emergency medical services, teaching life-saving techniques to communities, or engaging in public health initiatives, one truth remains constant: preparation and knowledge empower people to respond effectively in emergencies. This manual seeks to share that knowledge in a clear, concise, and accessible manner, making it an indispensable tool for all levels of experience.

The book is designed to cover a comprehensive range of first aid techniques. It starts with the basics, such as assessing the scene and ensuring personal safety, and progresses to advanced topics, including managing severe bleeding, cardiac emergencies, burns, fractures, and more. Special emphasis is placed on scenarios like choking, drowning, and trauma-related injuries, which demand immediate action. For professionals in high-stakes environments, sections on triaging multiple casualties and collaborating with emergency response teams provide valuable guidance.

This manual was crafted with the following goals in mind:

1. **Practicality**: Every technique and instruction in this book is evidence-based, field-tested, and

grounded in best practices. Visual aids and step-by-step instructions have been included to make learning straightforward.

2. **Accessibility**: Recognizing the diverse audience for first aid knowledge, the language has been kept clear and free of unnecessary jargon, without compromising on accuracy or depth.

3. **Inclusivity**: Whether you are a paramedic, firefighter, teacher, parent, or concerned citizen, this book offers life-saving skills tailored to your needs and capabilities.

4. **Empowerment**: By demystifying first aid, this book gives readers the confidence to act when it matters most, ensuring that more people feel capable of stepping in to save a life.

While this book draws from established guidelines and protocols, it also reflects my personal experiences in the field. Case studies and real-life examples have been incorporated to illustrate the practical application of the skills taught, helping readers understand the relevance and impact of each technique.

The urgency of learning first aid cannot be overstated. With preparation, you can make a profound difference in someone's life, often before professional medical help arrives. My hope is that **Essential First Aid Manual** will serve as both a learning tool and a quick reference guide in moments of need.

To those embarking on this journey, whether as first responders or members of the public seeking to make their communities safer, I commend your commitment. Your willingness to learn and act will not only save lives but also inspire others to do the same.

Thank you for trusting this book as your guide. Together, we can create a world where everyone is prepared to help in emergencies.

Sincerely,
Kyle M. Francois, EMT-P, MPH
EMS Educator and Public Health Specialist
National EMS Academy
2024

Introduction

First aid refers to the immediate care and assistance provided to an individual suffering from an injury or sudden illness. These interventions aim to stabilize the condition until professional medical help is available. In some cases, the situation may be minor, requiring only basic treatment and a calm, reassuring demeanor. Even minor injuries, such as cuts and scrapes, benefit from a sympathetic and composed approach as part of the care process.

However, certain accidents and illnesses can be severe or even life-threatening, where immediate action is crucial to prevent long-term disability, brain damage, or death. Procedures like cardiopulmonary resuscitation (CPR), which are discussed in this book, are life-saving techniques that require proper training. It is essential to learn and practice these skills under the supervision of a certified instructor, utilizing approved resuscitation manikins. Mastery of these techniques ensures confidence and precision during emergencies, significantly increasing the chances of saving a life.

Preventing accidents is equally important. Many injuries occur within the home environment, which is why this book includes a chapter dedicated to family safety. This section provides practical advice for making homes safer. Additionally, due to the prevalence of road traffic accidents, guidance is provided on managing emergencies at accident scenes. Emphasis is placed on accident prevention strategies, such as adhering to speed limits, avoiding driving under the influence, and practicing safe driving habits, which can protect both your life and others'.

How to Use This First Aid Book

This book is designed to be a straightforward, user-friendly guide for anyone seeking to learn first aid. It includes step-by-step instructions and a comprehensive A-to-Z reference of injuries and illnesses to ensure quick and efficient navigation, even in high-pressure situations.

The first section, Emergency, First Aid, and Safety Procedures, offers foundational knowledge for addressing critical medical emergencies such as unconsciousness, respiratory arrest, and cardiac failure. It also contains a chapter on handling road traffic accidents and provides essential tips for family safety, including assembling a first aid kit and understanding its application. Familiarizing yourself with this section ahead of time will prepare you to act effectively in emergencies.

The second section, A-to-Z of Injuries and Illnesses, is organized alphabetically to provide a quick reference guide for a variety of medical conditions, from common minor injuries to major health crises. This structure ensures that the information you need is accessible within moments, helping you respond promptly and appropriately.

By studying this book, practicing key techniques, and adopting preventive measures, you will be equipped to handle a range of emergency situations with confidence and competence.

Acknowledgement
Preface
Introduction
Table of contents
List of Abbreviations

Table of contents

Chapter 1: Emergency, First Aid & Safety Procedures

1.1 Preparation Before an Emergency
1.1.1 Familiarizing Yourself with First Aid
1.1. 2 Learning and Practicing CPR
1.1.3 Stocking First Aid Kits

1.2 Emergency Priorities
1.2.1 Recognizing Immediate Risks
1.2.2 Key Steps and Protocols (DRSABCD)

1.3 Responding to Emergencies
1.3.1 Safety and Scene Assessment

1.3.2 Effective Communication and Delegation
1.3.3 Dos and Don'ts for Casualty Care

1.4 DRSABCD Emergency Protocol
1.4.1 Danger Assessment
1.4.2 Response and Recovery Positions
1.4.3 Airway, Breathing, and CPR Steps

Chapter 2: Emergency Techniques

2.1 Assessing Unconsciousness
2.1.1 Recognizing Signs of Unconsciousness
2.1.2 Action Steps for Unresponsive Casualties

2.2 Airway Management
2.2.1 Clearing and Opening the Airway
2.2.2 Side Position Technique

2.3 Checking for Breathing
2.3.1 Observation and Physical Assessment
2.3.2 Initiating Rescue Breaths

2.4 Cardiopulmonary Resuscitation (CPR)

2.4.1 Adult and Child CPR Guidelines
2.4.2 Infant CPR Techniques

2.5 Rescue Breathing Techniques
2.5.1 Mouth-to-Mouth Resuscitation
2.5.2 Mouth-to-Nose and Mouth-to-Mask Methods
2.5.3 Infant-Specific Techniques

2.6 Importance of CPR Training
2.6.1 Hands-On Training and Proficiency

Chapter 3: Anatomy and Physiology: Understanding the Human Body Systems

3.1 Overview of Major Body Systems
3.1.1 Interdependence and Functionality

3.2 The Nervous System
3.2.1 Brain, Spinal Cord, and Nerve Functions
3.2.2 Trauma and Its Effects

3.3 The Cardiovascular System

3.3.1 Heart and Blood Circulation
3.3.2 Recognizing Circulatory Emergencies

3.4 The Respiratory System
3.4.1 Gas Exchange and Breathing Mechanics
3.4.2 Addressing Respiratory Obstructions

3.5 The Musculoskeletal System
3.5.1 Structural Support and Protection
3.5.2 Recognizing Spinal and Skull Injuries

3.6 The Urinary System
3.6.1 Waste Filtration and Excretion

3.7 The Endocrine System
3.7.1 Hormonal Regulation and Functions

Chapter 4: Road Traffic Accidents: Providing Immediate and Effective First Aid

4.1 Essential Safety Measures
4.1.1 Ensure Scene Safety
4.1.2 Signal and Alert Traffic

4.1.3 Secure Vehicles and Address Electrical Risks
4.1.4 Fire Safety Precautions

4.2 Administering First Aid
4.2.1 Casualty Assessment
4.2.2 Prioritize Care
4.2.3 Summon Emergency Services

4.3 Moving an Injured Person
4.3.1 When and How to Move a Casualty
4.3.2 Dragging Techniques
4.3.3 Human Crutch Technique

Chapter 5: First Aid Kits: Essential Components and Guidelines

5.1 General Guidelines for First Aid Kits
5.1.1 Labeling and Storage
5.1.2 Maintenance and Medication Management
5.1.3 Emergency Information
5.1.4 Accessibility and Safety

5.2 Home First Aid Kit Essentials
5.2.1 Basic Medical Supplies
5.2.2 Medications and Ointments
5.2.3 Specialized Tools
5.2.4 Bandages and Protective Items
5.2.5 Eye and Wound Care
5.2.6 Additional Essentials

5.3 Procurement and Certification

Chapter 6: Dressings, Pads, and Bandages: Effective Use and Practical Guidelines

6.1 Dressings
6.1.1 Purpose and Benefits
6.1.2 Key Considerations

6.2 Pads
6.2.1 Applications and Benefits
6.2.2 Specialized Pads: Ring Pad

6.3 Bandages

6.3.1 Types of Bandages
6.3.2 Application Techniques

6.4 Triangular Bandages
6.4.1 Versatility and Uses
6.4.2 Instructions for Folding

6.5 Roller Bandages
6.5.1 Purpose and Materials
6.5.2 Step-by-Step Application

Chapter 7: Slings: Purpose, Construction, and Application

7.1 Types of Slings and Their Purpose
7.1.1 Arm Slings
7.1.2 Elevation Slings
7.1.3 Collar-and-Cuff Slings

7.2 Steps for Applying a Sling
7.2.1 Positioning the Arm
7.2.2 Securing the Bandage Around the Neck
7.2.3 Stabilizing the Elbow
7.2.4 Tying the Sling

7.2.5 Securing at the Elbow
7.2.6 Monitoring Circulation

7.3 Key Considerations for Effective Sling Use

Chapter 8: Advanced First Aid Techniques

8.1 Managing Airway Obstruction
8.1.1 Recognition and Immediate Action
8.1.2 Heimlich Maneuver
8.1.3 Airway Adjuncts

8.2 Cardiopulmonary Resuscitation (CPR)
8.2.1 Adult CPR Techniques
8.2.2 Pediatric CPR Guidelines

8.3 Managing Severe Bleeding
8.3.1 Use of Pressure and Tourniquets
8.3.2 Hemostatic Agents

8.4 Handling Burns and Scalds
8.4.1 Classification of Burns
8.4.2 First Aid for Thermal Burns

8.4.3 Chemical and Electrical Burns

8.5 Managing Fractures and Dislocations
8.5.1 Identifying Types of Fractures
8.5.2 Immobilization Techniques

8.6 First Aid for Poisoning
8.6.1 Recognition of Symptoms
8.6.2 Immediate Actions Based on Poison Type

Chapter 9: Patient Examination

1. Introduction
1.1 Importance of accurate patient examination
1.2 Avoiding "tunnel vision"

2. Prioritize Safety
2.1 Assessing the environment
2.2 DRSABCD protocol

3. Systematic Body Assessment: "Nose to Toes"
3.1 Step-by-step injury evaluation
3.2 Addressing life-threatening conditions

4. Leverage Available Tools
4.1 Physical tools and sensory observations
4.2 Skin color and temperature insights

5. Collect Medical History: AMPLE Framework
5.1 Allergies
5.2 Medications
5.3 Past medical conditions
5.4 Last meal
5.5 Events leading to injury/illness

6. Vital Signs
6.1 Pulse assessment: normal ranges and technique
6.2 Body temperature monitoring

7. Medication Administration
7.1 Assisting with prescribed medications
7.2 Exceptions for asthma, severe allergies, and chest pain

8. Triage
8.1 Prioritizing injuries for treatment

9. Communication
9.1 Effective reporting to emergency services

10. Remote Area First Aid
10.1 Preparation essentials for remote locations

11. Post-Traumatic Debrief
11.1 Professional assistance for emotional recovery

Chapter 10: Managing Common Injuries and Illnesses

1. Asthma Attack
1.1 Pathophysiology and key symptoms
1.2 4x4x4 management protocol

2. Bites and Stings
2.1 Non-venomous animal bites
2.2 Snake bites: identification and management
2.3 Spider bites: funnel-web and red-back spiders

2.4 Marine animal stings: box jellyfish, blue-ringed octopus, and others

3. Key Warnings and Preventive Steps
3.1 Avoid harmful traditional interventions
3.2 Guidelines for specific emergencies

Chapter 11: Comprehensive and Professional First Aid Guide: Common Emergencies

1. Burns and Scalds
1.1 Definition and Causes
1.2 Signs and Symptoms
1.3 Immediate Actions

2. Chest Injuries
2.1 Overview
2.2 Fractured Ribs: Signs and Symptoms
2.3 Action Plan
2.4 Sucking Chest Wounds: Signs, Symptoms, and Actions

3. Choking

3.1 Partially Blocked Airway: Signs, Symptoms, and Actions
3.2 Completely Blocked Airway: Signs, Symptoms, and Actions

4. Concussion
4.1 Definition
4.2 Signs and Symptoms
4.3 Action Plan

5. Convulsions
5.1 Definition and Types
5.2 Febrile Seizures in Children
5.3 Epileptic Seizures

6. Cuts and Wounds
6.1 Minor Cuts and Abrasions
6.2 Stab Wounds and Embedded Objects

7. Diabetes
7.1 Overview
7.2 Hypoglycemia (Low Blood Sugar): Signs, Symptoms, and Actions

7.3 Hyperglycemia (High Blood Sugar): Signs, Symptoms, and Actions

8. Drowning
8.1 Overview and Prevention Measures
8.2 Immediate Action Plan

9. Drug Overdose
9.1 Signs and Symptoms
9.2 Immediate Action Plan

10. Electric Shock
10.1 Warning and Safety Precautions
10.2 Immediate Action Plan

11. Eye Injuries
11.1 Chemical or Heat Burns
11.2 Foreign Bodies
11.3 Black Eye

12. Fainting
12.1 Signs and Symptoms
12.2 Immediate Action Plan

13. Heat-Related Illnesses: Exhaustion and Stroke
13.1 Overview
13.2 Heat Exhaustion: Signs, Symptoms, and Management
13.3 Heat Stroke: Signs, Symptoms, and Management

14. Neck and Spinal Injuries
14.1 Overview
14.2 Signs and Symptoms
14.3 Management Precautions and Steps

List of Abbreviations

AED - Automated External Defibrillator

BLS - Basic Life Support

CPR - Cardiopulmonary Resuscitation

EMS - Emergency Medical Services

ETT - Endotracheal Tube

IV - Intravenous

JVD - Jugular Venous Distension

LOC - Level of Consciousness

MI - Myocardial Infarction

NPO - Nil Per Os (Nothing by Mouth)

O2 - Oxygen

PPE - Personal Protective Equipment

RLS - Rapid Life Support

SAMPLE - Signs & Symptoms, Allergies, Medications, Past medical history, Last oral intake, Events leading to the present illness/injury

SIDS - Sudden Infant Death Syndrome

SOB - Shortness of Breath

TBI - Traumatic Brain Injury

TIA - Transient Ischemic Attack

TQ - Tourniquet

V-fib - Ventricular Fibrillation

V-tach - Ventricular Tachycardia

WBC - White Blood Cells

Chapter 1
Emergency, First Aid & Safety Procedures

Preparation Before an Emergency

Familiarize Yourself: Take the time to thoroughly review the first aid techniques in this guide before any emergency arises. Preparation is key—don't wait until an accident or illness occurs.

Learn and Practice CPR: Master life-saving techniques like cardiopulmonary resuscitation (CPR). These skills are best learned through hands-on practice with a certified instructor, using approved training equipment. Confidence and accuracy in CPR can make the difference between life and death in critical moments.

Equip Yourself: Ensure you have well-stocked first aid kits at home, in your car, on boats, and while traveling. Refer to the First Aid Kits section for guidance on what to include.

Emergency Priorities

When someone is unconscious, their life may be at immediate risk due to potential airway blockages, cessation of breathing, or lack of circulation. Prompt action is critical.

Key steps include:

1. Immediate Action: Brain damage or death can occur rapidly without intervention.

2. Follow Protocols: Use the DRSABCD action plan systematically (outlined below).

3. Consult Guidance: Refer to the Emergency Techniques chapter for detailed instructions on each step of DRSABCD.

Remember During an Emergency

1. Safety First: Ensure the scene is safe for yourself, others, and the casualty before proceeding.

2. Stay Calm: While emergencies are stressful, maintaining composure and reassuring the casualty is crucial.

3. Time Matters: Every minute counts, so act swiftly.

4. Limit Movement: Avoid moving the casualty unless absolutely necessary for their safety.

5. Seek Help: Never leave the casualty unattended. Delegate someone to call for medical assistance. If alone, prioritize contacting emergency services as soon as possible.

6. Clear Communication: Provide emergency responders with concise details, including the

location, nature of the incident, number of people involved, and the extent of injuries.

7. No Food or Drink: Refrain from offering food or liquids to the casualty.

DRSABCD Emergency Protocol

1. Danger: Assess and eliminate hazards or relocate the casualty to safety if possible.

2. Response: Check if the person is conscious by asking simple questions or giving commands. Place unconscious individuals in a safe side position.

3. Send for Help: Contact emergency services immediately.

4. Airway: Ensure the airway is clear and unobstructed.

5. Breathing: Check for breathing. If absent, begin chest compressions.

6. CPR: Perform 30 chest compressions followed by 2 rescue breaths.

7. Defibrillation: Use a defibrillator if available, following the device's instructions.

Chapter 2
Emergency Techniques

Assessing Unconsciousness

Unconsciousness occurs when brain activity is disrupted, rendering the individual unable to respond or protect themselves. Signs include:

Lack of response to verbal or physical stimuli.

Inability to cough, swallow, or clear airway obstructions like saliva, blood, or vomit.

The tongue falling back and blocking the throat due to muscle relaxation.

Action Steps:

1. Assess Responsiveness: Ask questions like "What is your name?" or "Can you open your eyes?" Lightly nudge the individual, but never

shake them—especially infants or small children.

2. Position Safely: If unresponsive, place the person in the side (recovery) position and check for airway obstructions, breathing, and a pulse.

3. Monitor Continuously: If the casualty is breathing with a pulse, maintain the side position, ensuring the airway remains open. Regularly reassess until medical professionals arrive.

Side Position Technique

The side position, also known as the recovery position, ensures the airway stays clear and prevents complications from fluid obstruction.

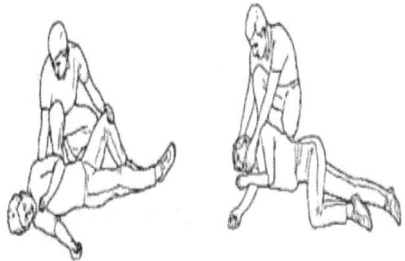

Steps:

1. Kneel beside the casualty.

2. Extend the arm farthest from you outward at a right angle to their body. Position the nearest arm across their chest, with the hand near the opposite shoulder.

3. Bend the nearest leg at the knee to form a right angle.

4. Gently roll the casualty onto their side by holding their shoulder and hip.

5. Adjust the top leg to rest on the ground, forming a stable position, with the thigh at a right angle.

6. Rest the bent arm on the straight arm for support. Tilt the head slightly back (for individuals older than one year), and angle the face downward to allow drainage and keep the tongue forward.

Clearing and Opening the Airway

The airway, which allows air to flow between the nose, mouth, and lungs, is essential for breathing. A blocked airway can immediately halt breathing, making it critical to ensure it remains clear and open.

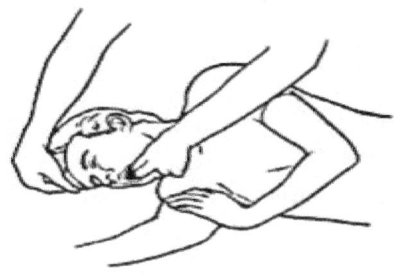

Steps to Clear and Open the Airway

1. Position the Casualty: Place the individual in the recovery (side) position to prevent airway obstructions.

2. Inspect and Clear the Mouth: Carefully examine the casualty's mouth for vomit, foreign objects, or loose or broken teeth. Remove obstructions with your fingers. Dentures should only be removed if they are damaged or unstable.

3. Open the Airway: To facilitate breathing, tilt the casualty's head back gently. Place one hand

on the forehead and use the other to lift the chin, ensuring the airway is unobstructed.

Checking for Breathing

Breathing should be smooth, quiet, and regular. Identifying irregularities quickly is vital in emergency situations.

Steps to Check for Breathing

1. Observe: Look for movement in the lower chest and abdomen, indicating respiratory activity.

2. Listen and Feel: Position your cheek near the casualty's nose and mouth to detect airflow.

3. Act if Necessary: If there are no signs of breathing, immediately begin chest compressions followed by rescue breaths.

Providing Rescue Breaths

Rescue breathing restores oxygen flow to the body when natural breathing has stopped. Mouth-to-mouth is the most common and effective method. In certain cases, alternative techniques such as mouth-to-nose or mouth-to-mask resuscitation are used:

Mouth-to-Nose: For casualties with severe jaw injuries or when in water.

For Infants and Small Children: Cover both the mouth and nose with your own mouth.

Mouth-to-Mask: Used by trained professionals to minimize contact and reduce the risk of disease transmission.

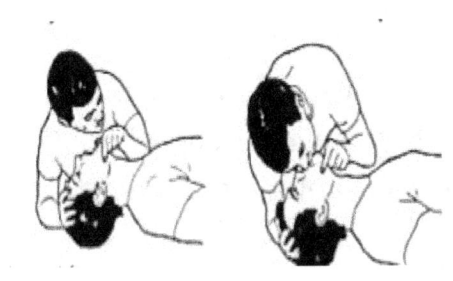

Steps for Mouth-to-Mouth Resuscitation

1. Position Yourself: Kneel beside the casualty to ensure stability.

2. Lay the Casualty Flat: Place the individual on their back for optimal access to the airway.

3. Tilt the Head and Open the Mouth: Gently tilt the head back, using your fingers to support the jaw without pressing on the throat. The casualty's mouth should remain slightly open.

4. Seal the Nose and Provide Breaths: Pinch the casualty's nose closed, take a deep breath, and seal your mouth over theirs to create an airtight connection.

5. Deliver Rescue Breaths: Administer two breaths, observing the chest for slight elevation. Avoid over-inflating the lungs.

6. Begin Chest Compressions: Follow the recommended compression-to-breath ratio.

7. Monitor Recovery: Once the casualty resumes breathing, place them in the recovery position and frequently reassess their airway, breathing, and pulse.

Cardiopulmonary Resuscitation (CPR)

CPR is a critical intervention for individuals in cardiac arrest, as it sustains circulation and oxygen delivery until advanced medical care becomes available. While two rescuers can alternate roles to maintain rhythm and reduce fatigue, even a solo attempt is better than none.

Adult and Child CPR

For adults and children, use a ratio of 30 compressions to 2 rescue breaths. Perform chest compressions at a rate of 100–120 per minute, focusing on the middle of the chest. Use the heel of one hand (or both hands for more force) to press down, ensuring the depth reaches one-third the chest's depth. Follow each set of compressions with two rescue breaths.

Infant CPR (Under 12 Months)

For infants, maintain the same 30:2 compression-to-breath ratio at 100–120 compressions per minute. Position two fingers in the center of the chest, between the nipples, and compress to a depth of one-third the chest's depth. Be especially gentle to avoid causing injury, as infants are more fragile. Follow compressions with two gentle rescue breaths, providing just enough air to make the chest rise.

Mouth-to-Nose Resuscitation

This technique is suitable when the casualty's mouth cannot be used due to injury or other circumstances.

Steps to Perform:

1. Position the casualty on their back and tilt the head back to maintain an open airway.

2. Support the jaw with your fingers, ensuring the mouth remains closed by sealing it with your thumb.

3. Take a deep breath, open your mouth wide, and cover the casualty's nose without compressing the nostrils.

4. Exhale into the nose, delivering enough air to cause chest rise.

5. Allow exhalation by moving your mouth away and opening the casualty's lower lip.

6. Repeat the process in alignment with the compression-to-breath sequence.

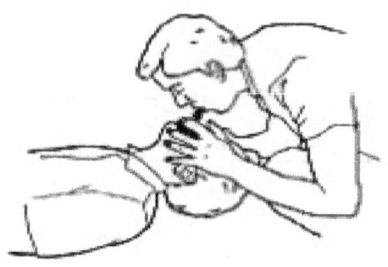

Mouth-to-Mask Resuscitation

Mouth-to-mask resuscitation reduces direct contact and is ideal when a mask is available, especially in cases of suspected infectious diseases.

Steps to Perform:

1. Position yourself at the top of the casualty's head, facing their feet.

2. Place the mask's narrow end over the casualty's nose, ensuring an airtight seal by pressing firmly with both hands while keeping the airway open.

3. Take a deep breath and exhale into the mask's mouthpiece, ensuring the chest rises visibly.

4. Allow exhalation by lifting your mouth from the mask.

5. Repeat the process as required, maintaining the recommended ratio of compressions to breaths.

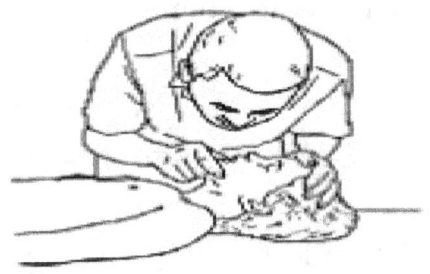

Mouth-and-Nose Resuscitation for Babies and Young Children

For infants and children under eight years old, mouth-and-nose resuscitation provides a practical approach to ensure effective ventilation.

Steps to Perform:

1. Clear the airway and position the child on their back. Slightly tilt the head if they are over one year old; keep the head horizontal for infants under one.

2. Create a seal by covering both the child's nose and mouth with your mouth.

3. Puff gently, delivering just enough air to make the chest rise slightly, avoiding excessive force.

4. Allow the child to exhale naturally, ensuring the airway remains open.

5. Repeat the sequence as needed, adhering to the compression-to-breath ratio of 30:2.

Importance of CPR Training

Although the techniques above provide essential guidance, hands-on CPR training is strongly recommended for proficiency. Rescuers trained through certified courses gain practical skills and confidence, enhancing their ability to respond effectively in emergencies. However, any attempt to perform CPR is better than none, and timely intervention significantly improves survival chances.

Chapter 3
Anatomy and Physiology: Understanding the Human Body Systems

The human body is composed of interconnected systems, each with specialized functions, yet dependent on one another to maintain optimal performance. When one system sustains damage, it inevitably affects others, emphasizing the interdependence of these systems. The major systems include the nervous, cardiovascular, respiratory, musculoskeletal, digestive, urinary, endocrine, lymphatic, reproductive, and integumentary systems.

The Nervous System

This system consists of the brain, spinal cord, and nerves, acting as the body's control center. The brain governs essential functions, while nerves transmit signals to and from different parts of the body. Any damage to the brain or the spinal cord—often caused by trauma to the skull or spinal column—can have significant consequences, including loss of motor or sensory functions.

The Cardiovascular System

Composing the heart, blood vessels, and blood, this system is responsible for transporting oxygen and nutrients throughout the body. Arteries carry oxygen-rich blood from the heart, while veins return oxygen-depleted blood. Blood loss from a severed artery can be rapid and life-threatening due to the heart's ability to circulate the entire blood volume in under a minute. Key pulse points, such as the neck, wrist, and groin, are critical for assessing circulation. If a pulse is absent, other indicators like skin color and temperature must be evaluated.

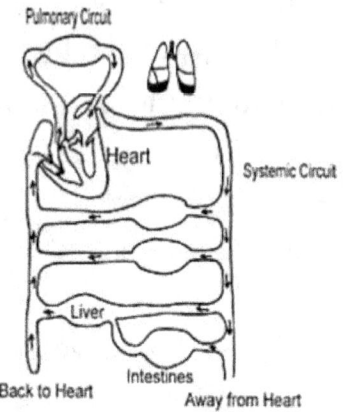

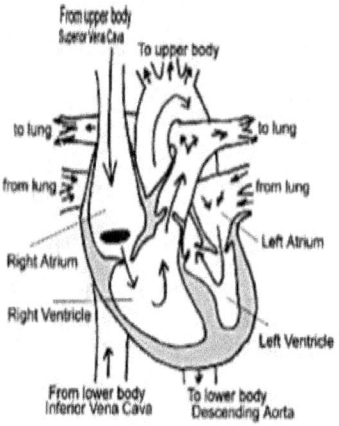

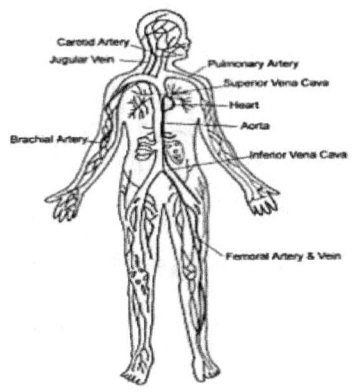

The Respiratory System

This system includes the mouth, nose, trachea, larynx, bronchi, bronchioles, and lungs. Its primary function is to facilitate gas exchange, delivering oxygen to the bloodstream while expelling carbon dioxide. A clear airway and proper breathing are essential for this process. If gas exchange is interrupted, the body quickly begins to suffer from oxygen deprivation, leading to critical conditions.

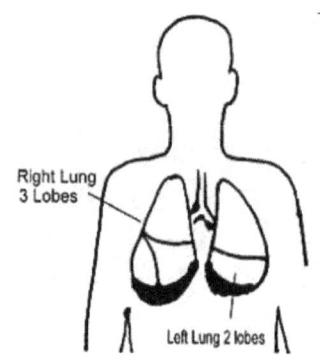

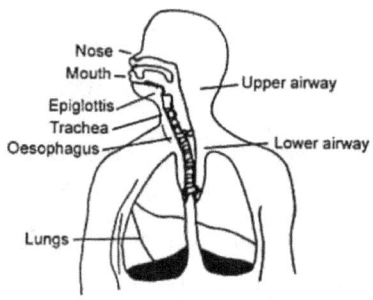

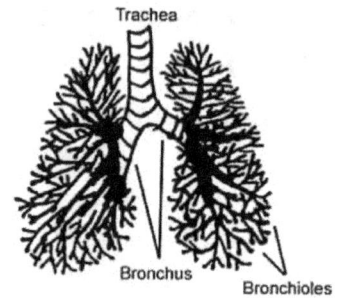

The Musculoskeletal System

The musculoskeletal system, made up of bones, muscles, tendons, and ligaments, supports body structure, enables movement, and protects vital organs. The spinal column not only supports the upper body but also shields the spinal cord. Injuries to the cervical spine are particularly severe and can result in conditions like paraplegia or quadriplegia. The skull, as part of this system, protects the brain from external impacts.

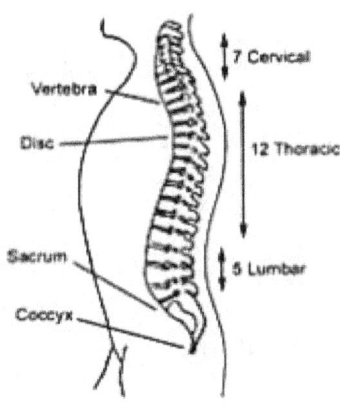

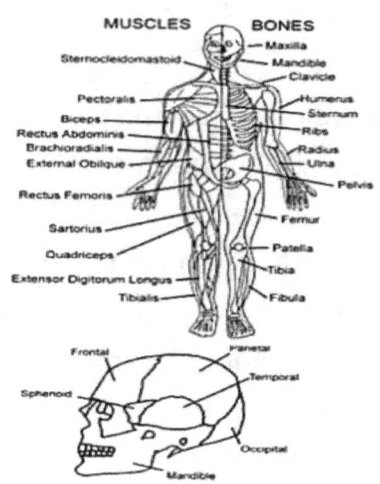

The Urinary System

This system includes the kidneys, bladder, and urinary tract, functioning to remove waste products dissolved in bodily fluids. By filtering blood and excreting waste, it maintains internal balance and overall health.

The Endocrine System

Through hormones, the endocrine system regulates bodily functions. For instance, insulin plays a crucial role in enabling cells to absorb glucose for energy. Disruptions in hormonal functions can lead to severe metabolic disorders.

The Lymphatic System

Often likened to the body's waste management system, the lymphatic system filters toxins and removes harmful substances. Its flow relies heavily on muscle movement. In cases of venomous bites or stings, applying a pressure immobilization bandage can slow venom distribution through the lymphatic system.

The Integumentary System

This system consists of the skin, hair, and nails, serving as the body's first line of defense against external harm, regulating temperature, and aiding in sensory perception.

The Reproductive System

Responsible for human reproduction, this system includes the organs necessary for procreation. It plays a vital role in the continuation of life.

The Digestive System

This system, encompassing the esophagus, stomach, and intestines, is tasked with breaking down food and absorbing nutrients for cellular energy and repair.

Importance of First Aid in System Damage

During emergencies, such as road accidents, immediate and effective first aid can prevent life-threatening complications. Quick intervention in the first few minutes can mitigate brain damage, heart failure, or severe blood loss. This highlights the importance of understanding human anatomy and physiology to provide life-saving care in critical situations.

Chapter 4
Road Traffic Accidents: Providing Immediate and Effective First Aid

Immediate and effective first aid at the scene of a road traffic accident can be life-saving. The first moments following an accident are crucial, as timely intervention can prevent fatalities from complications such as airway obstruction, cardiac arrest, or severe hemorrhage. Below is a systematic guide to ensuring safety and providing first aid during such emergencies.

Essential Safety Measures

1. Ensure Scene Safety

Confirm the scene is safe to approach, ensuring no hazards threaten rescuers or victims.

Protect yourself and others from oncoming vehicles by parking a vehicle as a barrier, if necessary.

2. Signal and Alert Traffic

Use hazard warning lights or flashing lights and, at night, low-beam headlights to increase visibility.

Place warning triangles or station individuals to signal oncoming traffic at a safe distance from the accident site.

3. Secure Vehicles and Address Electrical Risks

Switch off the ignition of all involved vehicles, engage the handbrake, and stabilize vehicles on inclines using wheel chocks.

Avoid contact with vehicles or casualties exposed to live electrical wires. Immediately notify electricity emergency services for assistance.

4. Fire Safety Precautions

Monitor for flammable substances, such as fuel leaks. Avoid smoking and have fire extinguishers ready for use if needed.

Administering First Aid

1. Casualty Assessment

Identify injured individuals, whether trapped in vehicles or on the roadside. Avoid smashing car windows unless the casualty is adequately shielded from potential harm.

Provide first aid to casualties in situ unless they are in imminent danger. For trapped individuals, adjust the car seat or other obstructions to relieve chest compression and ensure an open airway by tilting the head and supporting the jaw.

2. Prioritize Care

Focus on unconscious individuals first, assessing their airway, breathing, and circulation. Follow basic emergency protocols to address these priorities.

Control severe bleeding as soon as possible.

3. Summon Emergency Services

Contact emergency responders promptly, providing clear and concise information about the accident's location, the number of casualties, and the nature of injuries. Avoid leaving critically injured individuals unless absolutely necessary.

Moving an Injured Person

Moving a casualty should only be attempted when immediate hazards such as fire, traffic, or toxic fumes make remaining at the site dangerous. If moving is unavoidable:

Support the casualty's head, neck, and spine to prevent further injury.

Handle the casualty gently and move them smoothly, avoiding sudden movements.

Dragging Technique

When acting alone or in emergencies with severely injured or unconscious casualties:

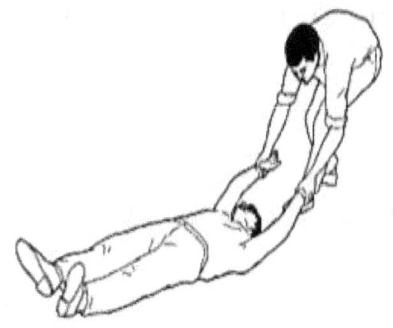

1. If there are no leg injuries:

Crouch at the feet, grip the ankles firmly, and gently drag the casualty backward.

2. If leg injuries are present:

Grip the elbows or wrists securely and proceed to drag the casualty backward, ensuring the body stays level with the ground.

Human Crutch Technique

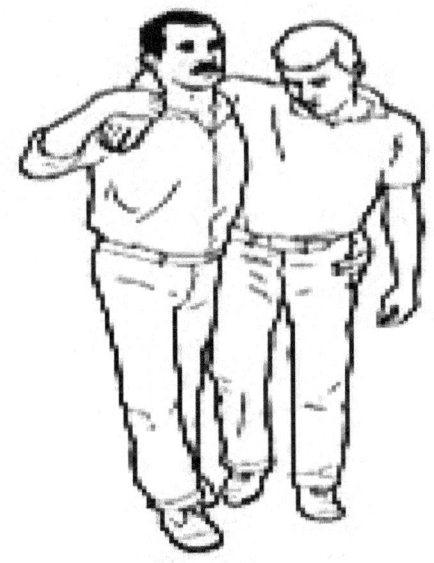

This method is suitable for assisting a conscious casualty who can walk with support:

1. Stand on the injured side unless the casualty's arm, shoulder, or hand is injured. In that case, position yourself on the opposite side.

2. Place your arm around the casualty's back, gripping their clothing at the far hip for stability.

3. Assist the casualty in placing their arm around your neck, supporting them with your shoulder. Hold their hand unless it is injured or bleeding.

4. Move forward together, coordinating steps to ensure balance and minimize discomfort.

Providing first aid during road traffic accidents requires a clear focus on safety, prompt assessment of casualties, and careful intervention. By adhering to these guidelines, rescuers can prevent further harm, stabilize victims, and improve their chances of survival until professional medical help arrives.

Chapter 5
First Aid Kits: Essential Components and Guidelines

A well-prepared first aid kit can significantly impact the outcome of medical emergencies by saving precious minutes. It's advisable to maintain a fully stocked first aid kit at home and carry additional kits in vehicles, boats, or during outdoor activities such as camping or traveling. Below are key guidelines and components to ensure your first aid kit is practical, safe, and accessible.

General Guidelines for First Aid Kits

1. Labeling and Storage

Clearly label the container with "First Aid" to ensure easy identification.

Use a durable, waterproof, and childproof container to protect the contents from damage or unauthorized access.

2. Maintenance and Medication Management

Replace used or expired items promptly to maintain readiness.

Dispose of leftover or expired medications responsibly. Never store medications for extended periods after completing prescribed courses.

3. Emergency Information

Attach a card to the kit listing emergency contact numbers, as well as information on blood groups, allergies, and specific medical conditions of family members.

4. Accessibility and Safety

Store the kit in an easily accessible location but out of children's reach.

Keep a reliable first aid reference guide close to the kit for immediate consultation during emergencies.

Home First Aid Kit Essentials

For a family setting, a comprehensive first aid kit should include the following items:

Basic Medical Supplies

Adhesive Dressing Strips: Useful for minor cuts and abrasions.

Adhesive Tape: For securing dressings in place.

Antiseptic Solution: To disinfect wounds and prevent infections.

Sterile Combine Dressings: Designed for severe bleeding.

Sterile Gauze Swabs: For cleaning wounds.

Sterile Non-Adherent Dressings: Ideal for burns.

Medications and Ointments

Paracetamol Tablets: For relieving minor pain and headaches.

Antihistamine Cream: To soothe bites and stings.

Specialized Tools

Disposable Latex Gloves: To maintain hygiene while providing care.

Splinter Forceps or Remover: For removing splinters safely.

Round-Ended Scissors: Designed specifically for cutting bandages and dressings.

Thermometer in a Protective Case: To monitor body temperature accurately.

Bandages and Protective Items

Roller Bandages: Available in various sizes to suit different injuries.

Triangular Bandages: Useful for slings or securing immobilized limbs.

Tubular Gauze Bandage with Applicator: Ideal for dressing fingers.

Eye and Wound Care

Sterile Eye Pads: Individually wrapped for eye injuries.

Cotton Buds: For precise application of antiseptic solutions.

Additional Essentials

Medicine Measure: For accurate dosing of liquid medications.

Safety Pins: To secure bandages or slings in place.

Procurement and Certification

To ensure quality and reliability, purchase first aid kits that meet regulatory standards, such as those approved by the Therapeutic Goods Administration (TGA).

A properly maintained first aid kit is indispensable in emergencies, providing the necessary tools to manage injuries effectively until professional help arrives. By following these guidelines and keeping the kit well-stocked, families can be better prepared to handle unexpected situations.

Chapter 6
Dressings, Pads, and Bandages: Effective Use and Practical Guidelines

The appropriate use of dressings, pads, and bandages is crucial for wound care and injury management. Each plays a unique role in controlling bleeding, preventing infection, supporting injured areas, and promoting recovery. Below is a detailed guide to their application and best practices.

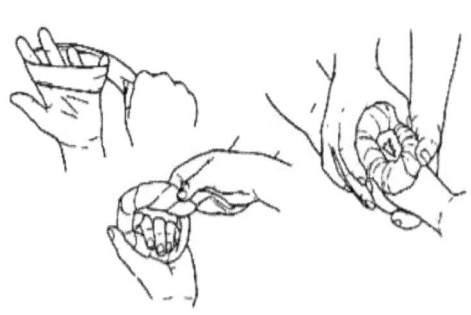

Dressings

A dressing is a sterile, protective layer applied directly over a wound. Its primary purposes include:

Controlling and Absorbing Bleeding: Helps manage fluid discharge.

Pain Relief: Provides a barrier that minimizes discomfort.

Infection Prevention: Shields the wound from contaminants and further injury.

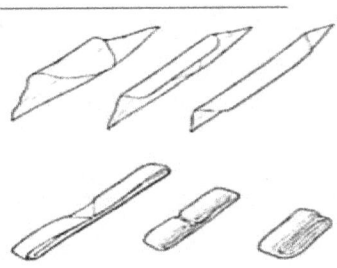

Key Considerations:

Use sterile, non-adhesive materials like gauze, linen, or specially designed dressings.

Avoid cotton wool or fluffy materials, as their fibers can adhere to the wound.

Refrain from touching the wound or any part of the dressing that will come into contact with the wound surface.

Pads

Pads are layers of cloth, gauze, or bandages used to:

Apply Pressure: Helps control bleeding and supports dressings.

Increase Absorption: Manages fluid discharge effectively.

Protect the Skin: Reduces irritation from bandages or friction.

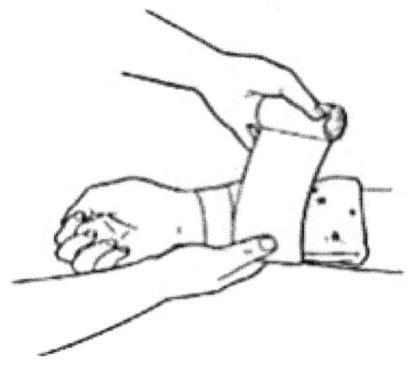

Specialized Pads: Ring Pad

A ring pad is particularly useful for wounds with embedded objects or protruding bones. It keeps the bandage elevated and away from the injury.

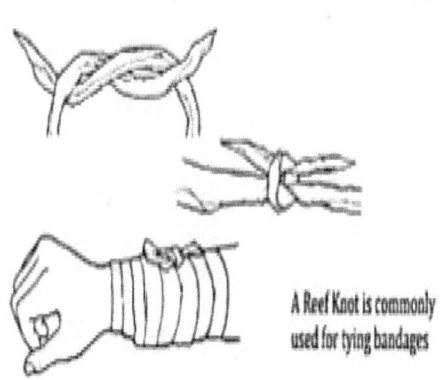

A Reef Knot is commonly used for tying bandages

How to Make a Ring Pad:

1. Wind one end of a narrow bandage around your fingers to form a loop.

2. Thread the other end through the loop.

3. Continue weaving over and under until the loop becomes firm.

Bandages

Bandages serve a variety of functions, including:

Controlling Bleeding by securing dressings in place.

Swelling Reduction through compression.

Support and Immobilization for injured limbs or joints, often in combination with splints.

Types of Bandages:

1. Modern Bandages:

Available in materials like crepe, elastic, or conforming gauze.

Easy to apply and effective in maintaining uniform pressure.

2. Tubular Gauze Bandages:

Convenient, as they don't require tying.

Designed for fingers, toes, and small areas.

3. Improvised Bandages:

In emergencies, use items like sheets, pillowcases, or stockings.

Important Notes:

Ensure bandages are not too tight. Signs of over-tightening include swelling, pale or bluish skin, numbness, tingling, pain, or absence of a pulse below the bandaged area.

Regularly inspect bandages for proper fit and circulation.

Triangular Bandages

Triangular bandages, typically made of calico or cotton, are versatile and commonly used to:

Secure large dressings or splints.

Create slings for arm injuries.

Protect areas such as the scalp, chest, or back.

Instructions for Use:

To Fold into a Narrow Bandage: Fold the triangle's tip to its base edge, then fold again. For a narrower bandage, repeat once more.

To Create a Pad: Fold both ends toward the center, then fold one half over the other.

Roller Bandages

Traditionally made of linen, cotton, or gauze, roller bandages provide consistent pressure and support.

Application Steps:

1. Position yourself opposite the injured person for better control.

2. Support the injured limb.

3. Hold the roll in one hand and apply the bandage outward from the body, starting below the injury and moving upward.

4. Overlap each turn by two-thirds, ensuring even pressure. Finish with two to three turns above the injury.

5. Secure the bandage by cutting and tucking the end or tying it with a reef knot.

Dressings, pads, and bandages are indispensable tools in first aid, providing critical support during emergencies. Proper application and regular monitoring are essential to ensure effective wound care, minimize discomfort, and facilitate recovery. Understanding these techniques enhances preparedness and improves patient outcomes.

Chapter 7
Slings: Purpose, Construction, and Application

Slings are essential in first aid for supporting, protecting, or immobilizing injured limbs. While commercial slings are available, they can be easily improvised using items such as triangular bandages, towels, pillowcases, or scarves.

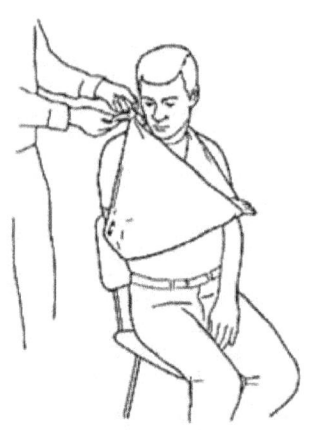

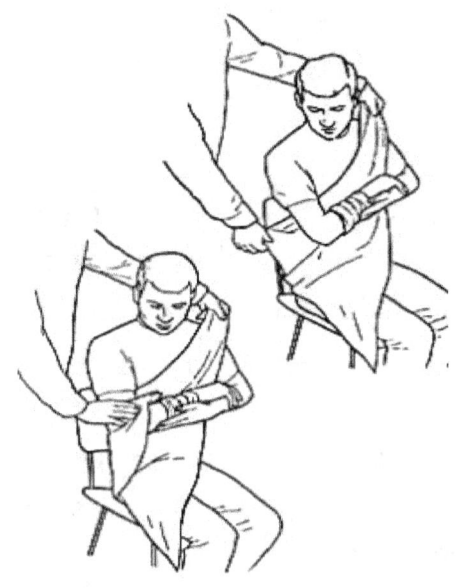

Types of Slings and Their Purpose

Arm Slings
Arm slings are commonly used to support an injured arm or an arm immobilized by a splint, such as in cases of forearm or wrist fractures.

Steps for Applying an Arm Sling

1. Position the Arm:

Ask the injured individual to hold their arm with the wrist and hand slightly elevated above the elbow. This helps reduce swelling and provides stability.

Place a triangular bandage between the arm and chest, ensuring the point of the triangle extends beyond the elbow.

2. Secure the Bandage Around the Neck:

Take the top end of the triangular bandage over the shoulder on the uninjured side.

Wrap it around the neck for proper support.

3. Stabilize the Elbow:

Fold the point of the triangular bandage around the elbow and tuck it securely between the upper arm and the sling.

4. Tie the Sling:

Bring the bottom end of the triangular bandage over the hand and arm, aligning it with the top end on the injured side.

Tie both ends into a reef knot in the hollow above the collarbone. This ensures a firm but comfortable fit.

5. Secure at the Elbow:

Use a safety pin to fasten the sling at the elbow fold for added stability.

6. Monitor Circulation:

Keep the fingernails visible and inspect them frequently.

If the nails appear blue or white, indicating restricted blood flow, loosen the sling slightly to restore proper circulation.

Key Considerations

Always ensure the sling is snug but not overly tight to avoid compromising circulation.

Check for signs of discomfort or changes in sensation, such as numbness or tingling, and adjust as needed.

If a sling is improvised, verify that the material used is strong enough to provide adequate support.

The proper application of a sling can significantly improve the comfort and safety of a casualty while minimizing further injury. Following these guidelines ensures effective support and immobilization, contributing to better outcomes in emergency care.

Elevation Sling and Collar-and-Cuff Sling: Proper Techniques and Uses

Both elevation and collar-and-cuff slings play essential roles in providing support and immobilization for specific upper limb injuries. Proper application not only reduces pain but also minimizes further injury.

Elevation Sling

Purpose:
The elevation sling supports the elbow while preventing strain on an injured shoulder. It is also effective for stabilizing a bleeding palm,

hand fractures, or injuries requiring elevation (e.g., to control bleeding).

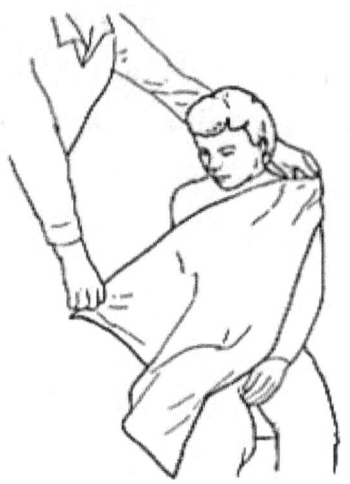

Steps to Apply an Elevation Sling:

1. Position the Arm:

Place the injured arm across the chest with the fingers pointing towards the shoulder on the injured side. This creates a natural elevation for support.

2. Position the Bandage:

Drape a triangular bandage over the forearm and hand, ensuring its point aligns with the bent elbow.

Place the top end of the bandage over the opposite (uninjured) shoulder and let the bass hang along the casualty's body.

3. Secure the Hand:

Hold the hand and the top end of the bandage resting on the uninjured shoulder.

Tuck the lower part of the bandage under the casualty's hand and wrist with your thumb, ensuring a snug fit.

4. Wrap and Tuck:

Use your free hand to tuck the triangular bandage's point under the upper arm.

Sweep your hand beneath the remaining section of the bandage and bring it up to secure the upper arm, folding any excess material neatly.

5. Tie and Secure:

Take the ends of the bandage around the casualty's back and tie them securely with a reef knot in the hollow above the uninjured collarbone.

Fasten the sling at the elbow fold with a safety pin to ensure stability.

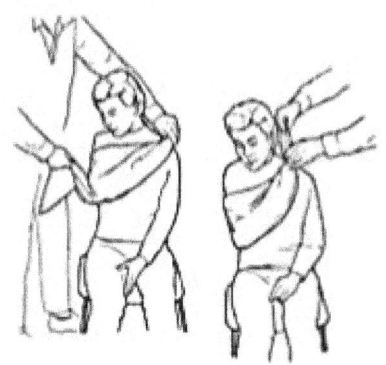

Collar-and-Cuff Sling

Purpose:
This sling is ideal for supporting an upper arm fracture (not near the elbow) or other upper limb injuries where wrist immobilization is unnecessary.

Steps to Apply a Collar-and-Cuff Sling:

1. Create a Clove Hitch:

Form two loops in the bandage, one facing you and the other away.

Slide the two loops together to create a secure hitch.

2. Position the Wrist:

Slip the clove hitch gently over the casualty's wrist on the injured arm. Ensure it is snug but not restrictive.

3. Support the Arm:

Position the casualty's forearm across the chest, allowing the fingers to point toward the opposite shoulder. Adjust the arm to a comfortable position for the individual.

4. Secure Around the Neck:

Take both ends of the bandage and guide them around the casualty's neck.

Tie the ends into a reef knot in the hollow above the collarbone, ensuring equal tension to avoid discomfort.

Key Considerations for Both Slings

Comfort: Ensure the sling is not too tight or loose, as either condition can compromise circulation or stability.

Circulation: Regularly check for signs of restricted blood flow, such as numbness, tingling, or discoloration of the fingers. Adjust as necessary.

Material: If a triangular bandage is unavailable, suitable alternatives such as scarves, ties, or belts can be used to create these slings effectively.

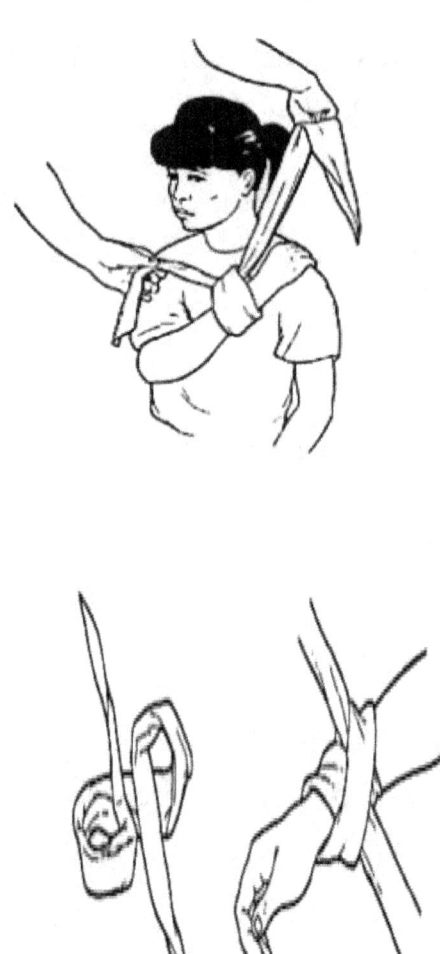

Properly applied slings, whether elevation or collar-and-cuff, are critical for managing upper limb injuries effectively. Following these steps ensures adequate support, minimizes pain, and protects against further injury while awaiting professional medical care.

SPLINTS

Splints are essential tools used to stabilize and protect injured limbs, particularly in cases of fractures. They immobilize the area to prevent further damage and support the healing process, especially when medical assistance is delayed. Splints can be used for fractures of the upper or lower leg, kneecap, upper arm, forearm, wrist, or fingers. While prefabricated wooden splints are readily available, improvisation with items like rolled newspapers or umbrellas can be effective in emergencies. In certain situations, such as a fractured femur, the uninjured leg can serve as a splint by securely bandaging the two legs together.

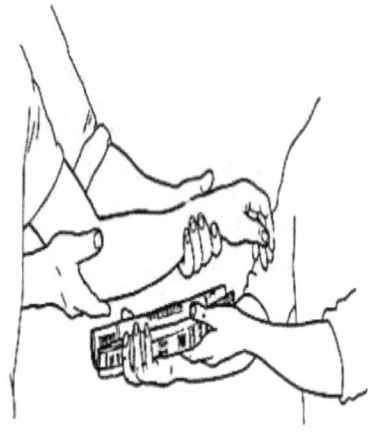

Key Considerations

Minimize Movement: Avoid unnecessary movement of the injured limb during splint application.

Appropriate Length: Ensure the splint extends beyond the joints above and below the fracture site.

Regular Monitoring: Check the tightness of bandages every 15 minutes to prevent restricted blood flow.

Clinical Judgement: If advanced medical help is available, allow professionals to manage splint application, as they can provide pain relief before immobilization.

Application Steps

1. Prepare Padding: Use clean materials, folded cloth, or bandages to cushion the splint. Pay special attention to bony areas such as the ankles and wrists.

2. Secure the Splint: Tie the splint firmly in place, ensuring stability without compromising circulation. Add extra padding to natural hollows for comfort and protection.

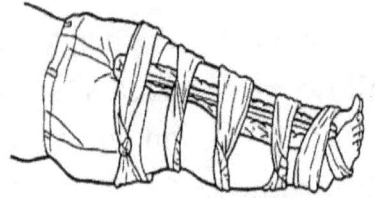

Chapter 8
Family Safety

The home environment can pose numerous safety risks. Each year in Australia, approximately 350 children die from preventable accidents at home, with countless others sustaining life-altering injuries. Elderly individuals and children are particularly vulnerable. Among household areas, the kitchen is the most hazardous due to the frequency of activities and potential dangers.

General Preventive Measures

Simple precautions can significantly enhance family safety. Below are area-specific checklists to mitigate risks and foster a safer home environment:

Kitchen Safety

Electrical Safety: Keep appliances and power points out of children's reach; use dummy plugs for low outlets.

Cord Management: Prevent appliance cords from trailing, especially near sinks or stoves.

Hot Liquids: Place teapots and hot drinks away from edges; avoid passing them over a child's head.

Knife Storage: Store knives securely.

Cleaning Products: Lock cabinets containing chemicals and store items like bleach and detergents out of children's reach.

Plastic Bags: Keep plastic bags away from children to prevent suffocation risks.

Cooking Safety

Use back burners when possible, turning pot handles inward.

Ensure children stay away from the stove; assign safe activities to keep them engaged.

Address spills promptly to prevent slipping hazards.

Take precautions with hot oil to prevent burns and fires.

Bathroom Safety

Double-check water temperature before bathing children, adding cold water first.

Keep all electrical devices away from water; use them in dry areas such as bedrooms.

Never leave children unattended in the bath; take them along if you need to leave.

Install non-slip mats and safety rails to prevent falls.

Store medications, razors, and cleaning supplies out of reach.

Garden Safety

Always wear gloves to protect against cuts and potential allergic reactions from spider bites.

Store garden tools and chemicals securely, ensuring proper labeling.

Avoid leaving children unattended near pools; empty wading pools after use.

Wear sturdy footwear while mowing or using electric tools.

Child Safety Measures

Prevent choking hazards by avoiding peanuts for children under three and supervising babies during meals.

Avoid using long ribbons for pacifiers; they can pose strangulation risks.

Ensure baby equipment meets safety standards, especially cots, high chairs, and strollers.

Use approved car seats and adjust safety belts appropriately for every trip.

Teach road safety and supervise children near traffic.

By following these detailed precautions, families can significantly reduce the risk of home accidents, ensuring a safer environment for all members.

Chapter 9
Patient Examination

Effective patient examination is a critical component of first aid, ensuring that the responder accurately identifies and addresses injuries. Misjudgment or "tunnel vision"—focusing only on obvious injuries—can lead to oversight of less apparent but significant conditions. Below is a structured, evidence-based approach to patient assessment:

Key Steps in Patient Assessment

1. Prioritize Safety

Before initiating treatment, assess the environment to ensure safety by eliminating potential hazards. This is crucial for the responder and the patient.

Adhere to the DRSABCD protocol: Danger, Response, Send for help, Airway, Breathing, Circulation, and Defibrillation.

2. Systematic Body Assessment: "Nose to Toes"

Begin at the head and proceed methodically to other body areas, checking for injuries such as cuts, swelling, abrasions, and bruises.

Address life-threatening conditions immediately, pausing further examination only to provide critical interventions. Comprehensive treatment should be deferred until the full assessment is complete.

3. Leverage Available Tools

Use both physical tools (bandages, slings, etc.) and sensory tools (visual inspection, touch to evaluate skin temperature or texture).

Observation of skin color and temperature provides additional insights into the patient's condition, complementing standard first-aid tools.

4. Collect Medical History Using the AMPLE Framework

A: Allergies

M: Medications

P: Past or present medical conditions

L: Last meal (important for potential surgical considerations)

E: Events leading to the illness or injury

Pulse Assessment

Although checking for a pulse is no longer part of CPR, it remains vital for evaluating conditions like shock or blood loss.

Normal Pulse Rates: Adults: 60–80 beats/min; Children: ≤100 beats/min; Infants: ≤140 beats/min.

Technique: Gently place two or three fingertips on the thumb side of the patient's wrist. Count beats for a full minute. If the pulse is difficult to locate, adjust finger placement.

Body Temperature Monitoring

Body temperature can indicate underlying issues such as shock, hypothermia, infection, or heat stroke.

Normal Range: 36.1°C–37.1°C.

Procedure:

1. Shake a mercury thermometer below 36°C.

2. Place it under the tongue, arm, or groin for three minutes.

3. For infants, use the armpit to avoid injury.

Medication Administration

First aiders must avoid prescribing medications but can assist in emergencies where patient-specific medications are already available. Exceptions include:

Asthma: Help administer Ventolin.

Severe Allergies: Assist with an EpiPen.

Chest Pain: Recommend a single aspirin, provided there's no allergy.

When in doubt, seek advice from emergency services or medical professionals.

Triage

Triage involves prioritizing patients based on the severity of their injuries. Even in minor emergencies, understanding which condition requires immediate attention ensures efficient use of time and resources.

Communication

Effective communication with emergency services must be concise and factual, avoiding speculation. Share key information, such as:

Injuries identified

Pulse rate

Skin color

Conscious state
This helps responders track the patient's condition over time.

Remote Area First Aid

Preparation is essential for providing first aid in remote areas. Ensure:

Adequate first aid supplies

Weather-appropriate clothing

Shelter-building materials

Sufficient water and communication devices
Consult local organizations for additional preparation tips.

Post-Traumatic Debrief

Experiencing traumatic events can affect individuals differently. Seeking professional assistance promptly after such incidents aids recovery.

Discussing the event with peers can provide initial relief, but professional guidance ensures proper emotional processing.

Remember, abnormal reactions to abnormal situations are normal.

This comprehensive, step-by-step approach ensures accurate patient assessment, timely interventions, and professional follow-up care.

Chapter 10
A Comprehensive Guide to Managing Common Injuries and Illnesses: Evidence-Based Approaches

Asthma Attack

Asthma is a prevalent chronic respiratory condition, particularly in Australia, where it affects approximately one in four children and one in ten adults. Individuals experiencing persistent symptoms such as shortness of breath, wheezing, or coughing should consult a healthcare professional for proper diagnosis and management.

Pathophysiology:
An asthma attack involves spasms of the bronchial muscles, swelling of the airway linings, and excessive mucus production, leading to airway narrowing and breathing difficulty.

Management:
Asthma patients should always carry a bronchodilator "reliever" medication, commonly delivered via metered-dose inhalers such as Ventolin, Bricanyl, or Respolin. The use of spacer devices significantly enhances the effectiveness of medication, especially in children.

Key Symptoms:

Difficulty breathing

Rapid, shallow breaths

Wheezing and coughing (often nocturnal)

Chest tightness

Difficulty speaking (severe cases)

Cyanosis (blue lips) and confusion in critical attacks

Warning:
Asthma can be life-threatening, requiring prompt action. If no medication is available, immediate medical attention is critical. Call an ambulance and specify the nature of the emergency.

Action Steps (4x4x4 Protocol):

1. Sit the patient in a comfortable, warm, and quiet environment.

2. Administer four puffs of the bronchodilator with a spacer if available.

3. Wait four minutes and repeat the dose if no improvement occurs.

4. If the condition persists or worsens, call for emergency assistance.

5. Continue administering the puffer as needed while awaiting medical help.

Note: Bronchodilator overdoses are rare during asthma attacks, and oxygen administration may be beneficial when performed by trained personnel.

Bites and Stings

Bites and stings can range from minor irritations to life-threatening emergencies, depending on the source and the individual's response.

Non-Venomous Animal Bites

Action Steps:

1. Clean the wound thoroughly with antiseptic or soap and water.

2. Apply a sterile dressing.

3. Seek medical attention for potential antibiotics, stitches, or a tetanus booster.

Snake Bites

Key Symptoms:

Puncture marks at the bite site

Redness, swelling, and pain

Nausea, vomiting, and headaches

Respiratory distress and unconsciousness in severe cases

Action Steps:

1. Immobilize the victim and avoid moving the affected limb.

2. Apply a pressure immobilization bandage.

3. Position the patient flat, avoiding limb elevation.

4. Administer CPR if necessary and call for emergency medical assistance immediately.

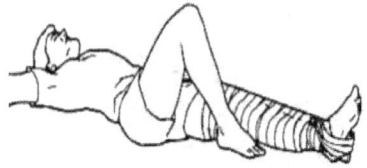

Warnings:

Do not cut, suction, or cauterize the bite.

Avoid using a tourniquet or washing the venom, as residue assists in identification.

Spider Bites (Funnel-Web and Red-Back)

Funnel-Web Spider:

Symptoms: Severe pain, nausea, breathing difficulties, and sweating.

Action: Treat as for snake bites and seek immediate medical help.

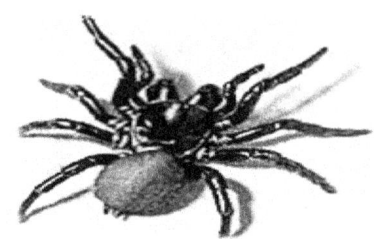

Red-Back Spider:

Symptoms: Localized pain, swelling, sweating, and potential shock.

Action: Apply a cold compress, monitor for shock, and seek urgent medical aid.

Marine Animal Stings (Box Jellyfish, Blue-Ringed Octopus, Cone Shells)

Box Jellyfish:

Symptoms: Intense pain, skin welts, difficulty breathing, and potential cardiac arrest.

Action: Douse the area with vinegar, avoid rubbing, and initiate CPR if necessary.

Blue-Ringed Octopus and Cone Shells:

Symptoms: Numbness, difficulty swallowing, and respiratory failure.

Action: Apply pressure immobilization and administer CPR as needed.

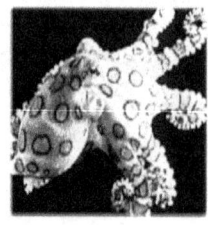 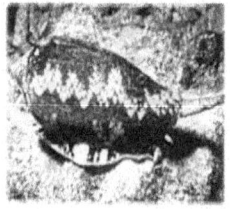

Other Stings (Stonefish, Stingrays, Blue Bottles)

Stonefish and Bullrout:

Symptoms: Intense pain, swelling, and potential shock.

Action: Soak the wound in hot water, remove any spines, and seek medical care.

Stingrays:

Symptoms: Immediate burning pain and respiratory distress.

Action: Avoid removing the barb, rinse with hot water, and monitor for breathing difficulties.

Blue Bottle Stings:

Symptoms: Severe pain from tentacle stings.

Action: Remove tentacles carefully, rinse with saltwater, and apply hot water.

Chapter 11
Comprehensive and Professional First Aid Guide: Common Emergencies

Burns and Scalds

Definition and Causes
Burns result from exposure to dry heat sources like flames, electricity, lightning, chemicals, and radiation (e.g., sunburn). Scalds, in contrast, are caused by moist heat such as boiling liquids or steam. Both are potentially life-threatening injuries, capable of causing infection, scarring, and, in severe cases, fatality.

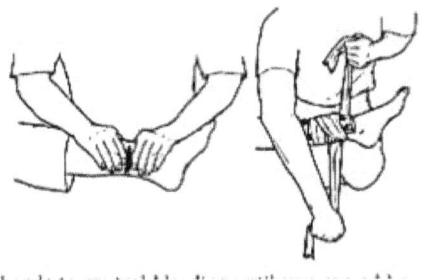

Signs and Symptoms

Superficial burns/scalds: Red, blistered skin; significant pain.

Deep burns: Dark red, blackened, or charred skin; absent pain if nerve endings are damaged.

Severe cases: Signs of shock, particularly with extensive burns or scalds.

Immediate Actions

1. Safety First: Remove the casualty from the heat source, ensuring your own safety.

2. Flame Suppression: If clothing ignites, smother flames using a blanket or rug. Avoid pouring water directly.

3. Unconscious Casualty: Place in the recovery position, check airway, breathing, and circulation (ABC), and initiate CPR if needed.

4. Clothing: Carefully remove burnt clothing unless adhered to the skin.

5. Cooling: Cool the affected area under running water (not icy) for a minimum of 10 minutes.

6. Dressing: Cover burns with a sterile, non-adherent dressing and secure lightly. Avoid ointments or creams.

7. Hydration: Offer water to sip if conscious. Avoid alcohol.

8. Rest and Elevation: Support burned limbs in a comfortable position.

9. Medical Attention: Seek immediate medical assistance for anything beyond minor burns.

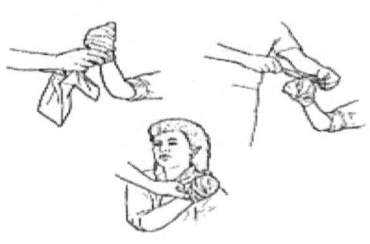

Chest Injuries

Overview
The chest contains vital organs such as the heart, lungs, and major blood vessels, making injuries to this area potentially life-threatening. Complications may include fractured ribs puncturing a lung, causing internal bleeding, or lung collapse due to air entering the chest cavity.

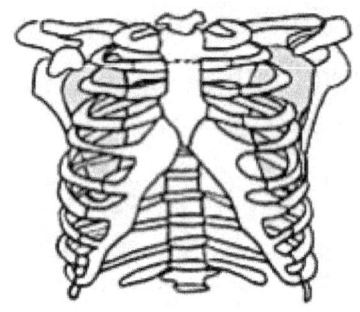

Fractured Ribs: Signs and Symptoms

Pain, exacerbated by breathing or coughing.

Breathing difficulties.

Frothy, blood-tinged sputum in severe cases.

Localized tenderness.

Action Plan

1. Unconscious Casualty: Place on the injured side, monitor ABC, and initiate CPR if required.

2. Conscious Casualty: Position in a half-sitting posture, leaning towards the injured side.

3. Padding: Place padding over the injury and secure it with a bandage.

4. Immobilization: Use a collar-and-cuff sling to stabilize the arm.

5. Emergency Care: Urgently seek medical aid.

Sucking Chest Wounds
Signs and Symptoms: Blood bubbling from the wound, bluish lips, difficulty breathing, and a characteristic sucking noise.

Action Plan:

Expose the wound and apply an airtight dressing taped on three sides to allow air to escape. Avoid completely sealing it.

Seek immediate medical help.

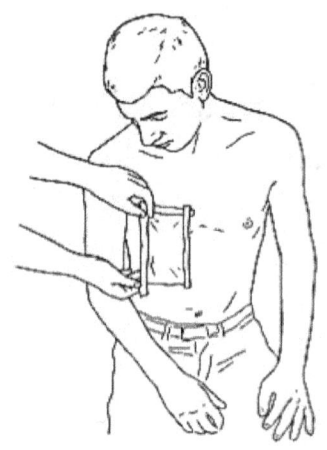

Choking

Partially Blocked Airway
Signs and Symptoms: Coughing, labored breathing, bluish skin, and possible unconsciousness.

Action Plan:

1. Encourage coughing if the casualty is able.

2. Avoid slapping the back unnecessarily.

3. If unconscious, place in the recovery position and seek urgent medical assistance.

Completely Blocked Airway
Signs and Symptoms: Inability to cough, breathe, or speak; chest not rising during rescue breaths.

Action Plan:

1. Position the casualty with the head lower than the chest.

2. Administer 3–4 back blows between the shoulder blades.

3. If ineffective, begin CPR and seek emergency help.

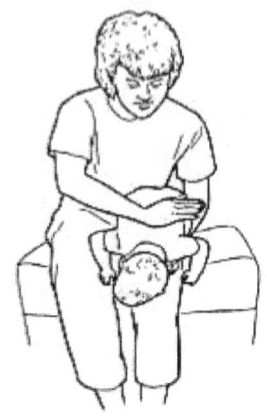

Concussion

Definition
A concussion is a temporary brain injury caused by a blow to the head, often resulting in a loss of consciousness or cognitive impairment.

Signs and Symptoms: Pale, clammy skin; shallow breathing; nausea; dizziness; short-term memory loss; and shock.

Action Plan:

1. Lay the casualty in a comfortable position. Avoid giving food or drink.

2. Apply a cold compress to the affected area.

3. Monitor for deterioration.

4. If unconscious, place in the recovery position and check ABC.

5. All head injuries with loss of consciousness require medical evaluation.

Convulsions

Definition and Types
Convulsions are caused by abnormal brain activity. Common causes include epilepsy, high fever (febrile seizures), and head trauma.

Febrile Seizures in Children

Signs: Jerking movements, limp body, breathing difficulties, and unconsciousness.

Action Plan:

1. Protect the child from injury but do not restrain them.

2. Place in the recovery position and keep the airway clear.

3. Remove excess clothing but avoid cooling with water.

4. Administer fever-reducing medication as directed by a physician.

Epileptic Seizures

Signs: Loss of consciousness, convulsions, frothing at the mouth, and temporary confusion upon recovery.

Action Plan:

1. Clear the area of hazardous objects.

2. Protect the head with a soft object but avoid restraining movement.

3. Post-seizure: Place in the recovery position.

4. Seek medical aid if the seizure lasts longer than 10 minutes or is the first occurrence.

Cuts and Wounds

Minor Cuts and Abrasions

Clean the wound with sterile water and antiseptic.

Apply a sterile dressing and seek medical aid if tetanus risk exists.

Stab Wounds and Embedded Objects

Apply direct pressure to stop bleeding.

Do not remove embedded objects; secure them in place with a ring pad.

Seek emergency medical attention.

Diabetes

Diabetes is a chronic condition characterized by insufficient or absent insulin production by the pancreas, leading to an inability to maintain normal blood sugar levels. Management involves dietary regulation, oral hypoglycemic agents, or insulin therapy.

Hypoglycemia (Low Blood Sugar):
When insulin levels exceed the body's needs or food intake is inadequate, blood sugar can drop significantly, causing unconsciousness.

Hypoglycemia is more common as an acute medical emergency than hyperglycemia, which usually develops more gradually.

Signs and Symptoms:

Dizziness or faintness

Hunger

Pale, sweaty skin

Tingling around the mouth

Rapid pulse

Slurred speech or confusion

Weakness

Possible unconsciousness

Immediate Action Plan:

1. Unconscious Person: Do not administer anything orally. Place them in the recovery position, ensuring their airway is clear, and monitor breathing and pulse.

2. Call for emergency medical assistance.

3. Conscious Person: Administer a sugar source like lemonade, orange juice, or water mixed with sugar.

4. Once symptoms improve, offer complex carbohydrates (e.g., fruit or a sandwich).

5. Advise consultation with a healthcare provider to identify the episode's cause and prevent recurrence.

Hyperglycemia (High Blood Sugar):
High blood sugar, if untreated, can lead to diabetic coma but typically progresses slowly, providing warning signs.

Signs and Symptoms:

Intense thirst

Frequent urination

Fatigue or drowsiness

Dry, flushed skin

Rapid pulse

Nausea, vomiting, or abdominal pain

Fruity-smelling breath

Possible unconsciousness

Immediate Action Plan:

1. If unconscious, position the individual laterally, ensure airway patency, and begin CPR if necessary.

2. Seek urgent medical assistance.

Drowning

Drowning occurs when water blocks the airway, leading to oxygen deprivation and potentially fatal outcomes. Rescue breaths should begin immediately, even before exiting the water if it is safe.

Prevention Measures:

Learn to swim and teach children to swim.

Never leave children unattended near water.

Learn basic rescue and CPR techniques.

Immediate Action Plan:

1. Remove obstructions from the airway and initiate mouth-to-nose rescue breaths if safe to do so in shallow water.

2. Once ashore, place the person in the recovery position and reassess the airway.

3. Begin or continue CPR as necessary.

4. Once breathing resumes, cover the individual with a towel or blanket to prevent hypothermia.

5. Seek immediate medical attention, as relapses are common.

6. Closely monitor the person's breathing and pulse until help arrives.

Drug Overdose

Drug overdoses, whether accidental or intentional, require prompt medical intervention.

Signs and Symptoms:

Dizziness or faintness

Seizures

Weak pulse

Breathing difficulties

Vomiting

Unconsciousness

Immediate Action Plan:

1. If unconscious, position laterally, ensure a clear airway, and begin CPR if needed.

2. If conscious, do not induce vomiting unless directed by a healthcare professional.

3. Identify the substance taken, and send relevant containers, syringes, or vomit samples with the patient to the hospital.

4. Call for emergency assistance immediately.

Electric Shock

Electric shock may range from mild tingling to cardiac arrest. Faulty wiring and improper use of appliances near water are common causes.

Warning:
Ensure your safety before assisting. Turn off the power source or, in high-voltage cases, wait for trained professionals to disconnect it.

Immediate Action Plan:

1. Use non-conductive materials (e.g., wood or rubber) to separate the victim from the power source.

2. Smother any flames on clothing.

3. If conscious, position the individual laterally and monitor airway, breathing, and pulse.

4. Treat burns and seek immediate medical help.

Eye Injuries

Eye injuries are serious and require immediate medical evaluation to prevent permanent damage.

Chemical or Heat Burns:

Signs: Pain, redness, swelling, and light sensitivity.

Action: Flush the eye with cool water for 20 minutes and cover with a sterile dressing. Seek urgent care.

Foreign Bodies:

Signs: Gritty sensation, redness, and irritation.

Action: Do not probe. Attempt gentle removal of visible objects using a moistened cloth or flush with clean water. Seek medical help if unsuccessful.

Black Eye:

Signs: Bruising and swelling from trauma.

Action: Apply a cold compress, avoiding direct contact with the eye. If swelling persists or vision is impaired, seek medical advice.

Fainting

Fainting occurs due to a temporary reduction in blood flow to the brain, often triggered by heat, exhaustion, or emotional stress.

Signs and Symptoms:

Pale, clammy skin

Weak pulse

Dizziness or blurred vision

Temporary unconsciousness

Immediate Action Plan:

1. Lay the person flat with legs elevated.

2. Loosen tight clothing and ensure fresh air circulation.

3. Check breathing and pulse.

4. Allow recovery before assisting the person to stand. Seek medical evaluation if consciousness doesn't return promptly.

Heat-Related Illnesses: Exhaustion and Stroke

Overview
Hyperthermia encompasses conditions such as heat exhaustion and heat stroke. Heat exhaustion results from significant fluid loss through sweating, whereas heat stroke is a critical medical emergency caused by the failure of the body's thermoregulatory mechanisms. Immediate recognition and intervention are vital to prevent complications.

Heat-related illnesses are more likely in hot, humid environments, particularly during prolonged physical activity. Vulnerable populations, such as infants and the elderly, face heightened risks due to less efficient body temperature regulation. For instance, leaving an infant in a closed car on a hot day can rapidly lead to hyperthermia.

Heat Exhaustion

Signs and Symptoms

Persistent feelings of heat and fatigue

Headache and dizziness

Thirst, nausea, and muscle cramps

Cool, clammy, pale skin with heavy sweating

Accelerated pulse and breathing

Disorientation and irritability

Management Steps

1. Move the individual to a cooler, well-ventilated space.

2. Position them supine and loosen or remove unnecessary clothing.

3. Apply cool water to their skin using a sponge or damp cloth.

4. Encourage gradual hydration with water or a diluted glucose solution.

5. Use ice packs on cramped muscles if applicable.

6. If symptoms persist or vomiting occurs, seek urgent medical attention.

Heat Stroke

Signs and Symptoms

Hot, dry, and flushed skin

Severe headache and dizziness

Body temperature exceeding 40°C (104°F)

Rapid, forceful heartbeat

Nausea, vomiting, and confusion

Possible loss of consciousness

Management Steps

1. If unconscious, position the individual laterally, ensure airway patency, and initiate CPR if necessary.

2. Relocate them to a shaded, cool environment.

3. Remove excess clothing and apply ice packs to the neck, groin, and armpits. Wrap them in a damp sheet and use a fan to expedite cooling.

4. Immediately contact emergency medical services.

5. Monitor body temperature every five minutes, ceasing cooling measures once the skin feels cool.

6. Upon regaining consciousness, administer small sips of fluid as tolerated.

Neck and Spinal Injuries

Overview
Suspected spinal injuries necessitate utmost caution to avoid exacerbating damage, which may lead to paralysis or respiratory failure. Such injuries often coincide with unconsciousness following head trauma.

Signs and Symptoms

Intense pain or tenderness at the injury site

Tingling in extremities and loss of movement or sensation

Severe cases may exhibit bowel/bladder incontinence and breathing difficulties

Management Precautions

Avoid moving the individual unless safety demands it.

Support the head, neck, and spine during movement if necessary.

Management Steps

1. If unconscious, use the lateral position while stabilizing the head and neck. Ensure breathing and pulse are present and perform CPR if needed.

2. Keep a conscious individual still and covered. Avoid raising the head or offering food/drink.

3. Seek urgent medical intervention.

Nosebleeds

Overview
Nosebleeds commonly arise from trauma, excessive nose-blowing, or high blood pressure. In rare cases, they may signal a severe head injury if accompanied by pale fluid leakage.

Management Steps

1. Advise the individual to breathe through their mouth and avoid nose-blowing.

2. Have them sit down, lean forward slightly, and pinch their nostrils for 10 minutes.

3. Loosen tight clothing around the neck and chest.

4. If bleeding persists, repeat the process or seek medical advice.

Hypothermia

Overview
Hypothermia, marked by extreme body cooling, occurs due to prolonged exposure to cold, wet, or windy conditions. Contributing factors include immersion in cold water and impaired thermoregulation caused by alcohol or drugs.

Signs and Symptoms
Mild to Moderate Cases:

Persistent shivering, fatigue, and reduced alertness

Slurred speech, poor coordination, and drowsiness

Severe Cases:

Cold, pale skin; shallow breathing; and slow pulse

Unconsciousness, particularly in infants or the elderly

Management Precautions

Avoid sudden rewarming to prevent shock.

Do not use direct heat sources like heaters or hot water bottles.

Management Steps

1. For mild cases, replace wet clothing with warm, dry layers, and offer warm fluids if conscious.

2. For severe cases, prioritize gradual rewarming and seek immediate medical assistance.

Frostbite

Overview
Frostbite occurs when blood flow to extremities diminishes, leading to tissue damage. Severe cases may result in gangrene and require amputation.

Signs and Symptoms

Tingling, numbness, and firm, waxy skin

Pain upon rewarming and the formation of blisters

Management Precautions

Do not rub affected areas or apply direct heat.

Management Steps

1. Move to a warm, dry environment.

2. Warm the area gradually using body heat.

3. Cover blisters with sterile dressings and seek medical care.

Poisoning

Overview

Poisons may enter the body through ingestion, inhalation, absorption, or injection. Timely identification and management are crucial.

Signs and Symptoms

Pain, nausea, vomiting, or difficulty breathing

Fainting, confusion, or unconsciousness

Burns in or around the mouth

Management Steps

1. For unconscious individuals, position laterally and perform CPR if necessary.

2. For conscious individuals, identify the poison and treat accordingly. Avoid inducing vomiting unless instructed by a professional.

3. Contact the Poison Control Center or seek emergency care.

Special Considerations

Corrosives: Rinse the mouth without inducing vomiting.

Inhaled Poisons: Ensure ventilation and avoid inhaling fumes yourself.

Absorbed Poisons: Remove contaminated clothing and wash skin thoroughly.

SHOCK

Shock is a critical, life-threatening medical condition caused by inadequate blood flow and oxygen delivery to tissues. It may result from intense pain, substantial blood loss, or excessive fluid loss due to severe injuries, burns, vomiting, or diarrhea. Shock progresses rapidly and requires close observation, especially following an accident or sudden illness.

Key Indicators of Shock

Pale, cold, and clammy skin

Weak, rapid pulse

Accelerated breathing

Lightheadedness or dizziness

Nausea

Thirst

Restlessness or agitation

Drowsiness and confusion, which may progress to unconsciousness

Management Steps

1. Unconscious Casualty:

Position the individual in the recovery position.

Ensure airway patency and monitor breathing and pulse.

Initiate CPR if necessary.

2. Conscious Casualty:

Lay the individual flat on their back.

Identify and address the underlying cause, such as bleeding, burns, or cardiac events.

3. Call for emergency medical assistance immediately.

4. Loosen restrictive clothing and help maintain body temperature without overheating the individual.

5. Refrain from giving food or drink; if the casualty is thirsty, wet their lips instead.

6. Regularly monitor airway, breathing, and circulation.

SPLINTERS

Even small splinters can cause infections if not removed properly. Deeply embedded splinters should be treated by a medical professional.

Procedure for Splinter Removal

1. Sterilize tweezers or splinter removers by boiling them for five minutes or exposing them to a flame.

2. Wash the affected area thoroughly.

3. Use tweezers to grip the splinter close to the skin and gently pull it out. If the splinter is difficult to access, use a splinter remover.

4. Clean the wound with mild antiseptic and apply a sterile adhesive dressing if needed.

5. Seek medical help if the wound shows signs of infection or swelling.

SPRAINS AND DISLOCATIONS

Sprains

A sprain occurs when a ligament is overstretched or torn, often due to joint overextension.
Symptoms:

Pain and tenderness around the joint

Swelling and bruising

Limited joint mobility

Management:

1. Apply a compression bandage to stabilize the joint.

2. Rest the joint and use ice packs to reduce swelling and pain.

3. Seek medical evaluation.

Dislocations

Dislocation involves displacement of bones in a joint, frequently occurring in the shoulder, elbow, or jaw.
Symptoms:

Severe pain

Visible deformity

Swelling and immobility

Management:

1. Immobilize the joint in a comfortable position.

2. Apply ice to reduce swelling.

3. Do not attempt to reposition the joint manually.

4. Seek immediate medical attention.

STRAINS

Strains result from overstretching muscles or tendons, commonly during physical activities or falls.

Symptoms:

Sudden, sharp pain

Increased discomfort with movement

Tenderness and reduced muscle strength

Management:

1. Rest the injured area and support the limb.

2. Apply ice packs to reduce inflammation.

3. Avoid massaging the affected area; instead, apply a firm bandage.

4. Gradual, gentle exercise may relieve muscle spasms.

5. Consult a healthcare provider if pain persists.

STROKE

A stroke results from interrupted blood supply to the brain, often due to arterial blockages or ruptures.

Symptoms (use FAST for early recognition):

Facial drooping

Arm weakness

Speech difficulty

Time to seek help urgently

Management:

1. If unconscious, place the person in the recovery position, ensuring an open airway and regular breathing.

2. Seek immediate medical assistance.

3. For conscious individuals, prop them upright with pillows, loosen restrictive clothing, and keep them warm.

SUNBURN

Prolonged exposure to strong sunlight can result in painful skin damage, including redness, swelling, and blistering.

Prevention:

Avoid sun exposure during peak hours.

Use protective clothing, hats, and sunscreen with high SPF.

Management:

1. Move the person to a shaded area or indoors.

2. Soothe the affected area with cool compresses or a shower.

3. Provide ample fluids to prevent dehydration.

4. Avoid popping blisters.

5. Seek medical advice for severe cases or for children with significant burns.

SWALLOWED OBJECTS

Small objects often pass through the digestive system without issues, but sharp or large items require urgent care.

Management:

1. Do not provide food or drinks.

2. Transport the individual to a medical facility promptly.

Teeth Injuries

Knocked-out teeth can often be saved if immediate action is taken.

Management:

1. Rinse the tooth with saliva, milk, or clean water.

2. Attempt to reposition the tooth in its socket, holding it there for at least two minutes.

3. If replacement is not possible, store the tooth in milk or saliva.

4. Seek dental care immediately.

Vomiting and Diarrhea

These symptoms can lead to dehydration and are often caused by viral infections or food poisoning.

Dehydration in Children:

Dry mouth

Sunken eyes

Lethargy

Management:

1. Provide oral rehydration fluids, starting with small, frequent sips.

2. Gradually reintroduce solid foods after 24 hours.

3. Seek medical attention for severe or persistent symptoms.

QUICK CPR QUIZ

1. Correct First Aid Acronym: DRSABCD

2. CPR Ratio: 30:2

3. Compressions per Minute: 100–120

4. Correct Hand Position: Middle of the chest

5. Perform CPR on Breathing Patient?: No

6. Use Defibrillator in Cardiac Arrest?: Yes

7. CPR Criteria: Unconscious and absent breathing

References

1. American Heart Association. (2020). Basic Life Support Provider Manual. Dallas, TX: American Heart Association.

2. World Health Organization. (2019). First Aid Guidelines: Essential Emergency Care for Communities and Providers. Geneva, Switzerland: WHO Press.

3. Tintinalli, J. E., Ma, O. J., & Yealy, D. M. (2020). Tintinalli's Emergency Medicine: A Comprehensive Study Guide (9th ed.). New York, NY: McGraw Hill.

4. St. John Ambulance. (2018). First Aid Manual: The Authorized Guide to Emergency Procedures (11th ed.). London, UK: Dorling Kindersley.

5. American Red Cross. (2019). First Aid/CPR/AED Participant's Manual. Washington, DC: American Red Cross.

6. Bergeron, J. D., Le Baudour, C., & Keith, K. (2017). First Aid for Emergency Care (7th ed.). Boston, MA: Pearson.

7. Porth, C. M. (2014). Essentials of Pathophysiology: Concepts of Altered Health States (4th ed.). Philadelphia, PA: Wolters Kluwer Health.

8. Wylie, P., & Churchill-Davidson, H. (2019). A Practice of Anesthesia for Infants and Children (6th ed.). Philadelphia, PA: Elsevier.

9. National Association of Emergency Medical Technicians (NAEMT). (2021). PHTLS: Prehospital Trauma Life Support (9th ed.). Burlington, MA: Jones & Bartlett Learning.

10. Smith, K. E., & Parker, R. (2018). Trauma Nursing: From Resuscitation Through

Rehabilitation (5th ed.). St. Louis, MO: Mosby Elsevier.

www.ingramcontent.com/pod-product-compliance
Lightning Source LLC
Chambersburg PA
CBHW071025240526
45469CB00006BD/2094